Zoilo Emilio Luna Tarazona

Yopo: Chemical Analysis and its implications in Forensic Toxicology

Zoilo Emilio Luna Tarazona

Yopo: Chemical Analysis and its implications in Forensic Toxicology

Case: Death of indigenous Yanomami people

ScienciaScripts

Imprint
Any brand names and product names mentioned in this book are subject to trademark, brand or patent protection and are trademarks or registered trademarks of their respective holders. The use of brand names, product names, common names, trade names, product descriptions etc. even without a particular marking in this work is in no way to be construed to mean that such names may be regarded as unrestricted in respect of trademark and brand protection legislation and could thus be used by anyone.

Cover image: www.ingimage.com

This book is a translation from the original published under ISBN 978-613-9-40702-6.

Publisher:
Sciencia Scripts
is a trademark of
Dodo Books Indian Ocean Ltd. and OmniScriptum S.R.L publishing group

120 High Road, East Finchley, London, N2 9ED, United Kingdom
Str. Armeneasca 28/1, office 1, Chisinau MD-2012, Republic of Moldova, Europe
Printed at: see last page
ISBN: 978-620-6-45140-2

GENERAL INDEX

INTRODUCTION

The concern or motivation to perform this work, arose based on a forensic case, related to an event that occurred in Puerto Ayacucho, capital of Amazonas state, Venezuela, in 2015. In which a member of the Yanomami people lost his life and involved members of the Municipal Police of the locality or territorial entity. The case was under the competence of the Prosecutor's Office against the Violation of Fundamental Rights, as well as those that protect the rights of indigenous peoples, embodied in the current Organic Law of Indigenous Peoples and Communities (year 2005).

In addition to the inquiry for police excess towards this security body of the State, the fact that the victim did not observe a rule, being under the effects of a psychoactive substance in the public street, as a consequence, his conduct was not conscientious, was also aired, Following this behavioral pattern, the police commission that approached the individual showed that they had no orientation or training to coordinate and provide a solution to this type of situation, and tried to subdue the Indian by applying brute and excessive force.(Art.19-21 of the Constitution of the Bolivarian Republic of Venezuela, 1999).

Since it is a violent event in which a citizen dies, a series of actions must be carried out that are the responsibility of both Criminalistics and Forensic Sciences, in order to determine the fatal injuries suffered by this member of the Yanomami people, in addition to collecting organic samples, particularly biological fluids of the deceased, to detect through a toxicological expertise, what type of substance or chemical agent the person consumed at the time of the event to be investigated.

However, they encountered a limitation, the Yanomami people among their customs and cosmogonic beliefs, do not contemplate performing autopsies of any kind (legal or clinical), they inhume their fellow human beings, then when they consider it convenient, they exhume the remains and with these they prepare a kind of soup or broth, which when ingested, according to Aparicio et al, (2015) they hope that the spirit of the deceased reaches the desired plane of existence, which entails immortality, happiness and the maintenance of the natural order of the universe, as well as agreements, alliances, both political and commercial. This spiritual-material duality that emerges from the funeral ritual in the practice of endocannibalism, constitutes the true socio-cultural essence of the Yanomami people.

It should be noted that this is called endocannibalism or funerary cannibalism by social anthropologists such as Lizot, (2007), Zucchi, (2000), as well as other experts and scholars of native peoples. Since the meat or substances to be ingested are obtained from the bodies of the deceased, who belong to the group itself, if it were from another group or people, it is only called cannibalism. Within the cultural system of the Yanomami people, funeral rituals are articulated as a complex practice through which the society of this native people establishes a connection between various aspects related to their beliefs about life and death (Aparicio et al., 2015). It is important that Western civilization develops enough tolerance and intelligence to understand the cultural meaning of death for the Yanomami people and not to consider it as a barbarism, incurring in disrespect to this ancestral culture.

After overcoming the above mentioned limitation, in addition to continuing with the due process, another limitation arises, the forensic laboratories of the Metropolitan Area of Caracas, which were requested to perform the toxicological analysis of the biological samples, according to information provided by the Prosecutor's Office leading the investigation, rejected the request, since they did not have a pattern of Di-methyltryptamine (active principle of yopo) or its metabolites, to compare against the results of the forensic toxicological analysis.

As a last resort, the Prosecutor's Office in charge of the case, requested the support of the Criminalistic Unit Against the Violation of Fundamental Rights of the Metropolitan Area of Caracas (UCCVDF-AMC), which has a Criminalistic Laboratory, and the request for expertise was sent to the area of Forensic Toxicology, attached to the Forensic Sciences Division of the aforementioned Unit. Which lacked a standard of Di-methyltryptamine or its metabolites, to compare the results, which would provide the relevant analytical tests, of the physical evidence in question (blood and gastric content).

For this reason, the author of this research, the expert responsible for the toxicological analysis (Forensic Toxicology Area of the UCCVDF-AMC), promoted an experimental work, to develop an internal pattern of the hallucinogen already mentioned. For this, it was first necessary to have the seeds of the Amazonian plant commonly known as yopo, whose binomial name is Anadenanthera peregrina (described and classified by the Italian botanist Carlos Luis Spegazzini, 1923) or Piptadenia peregrina (described and classified by the English botanist George Bentham, 1841; as well as by the also English botanist John Patrick Micklethwait Brenam, 1955), and on the other hand to determine which analytical methods would be the most suitable for the diagnosis of the presence of the alkaloid.

The objective of the forensic toxicological analysis, particularly in this case, is pragmatic, to detect in the collected samples (blood and gastric content), traces of dimethyltryptamine (yopo) or, failing that, any other substance that could be under the restriction of a regulation (Organic Law on Drugs, 2011) and that the results of this expert report will be useful to all the entities that administer justice (Courts, Public Prosecutor's Office, Public Defender's Office), as well as to the Criminal Investigation Corps, in order to carry out a suitable work.

To achieve the extraction of the active principle that concerns us in this case, the seeds from the plant called yopo (Piptadenia / Anadenanthera peregrina), were subjected to a relevant analytical march. In the same way, the biological fluid (blood), collected during the medico-legal autopsy of the Yanomami Indian's body, was processed in order to verify if the victim consumed any psychoactive substance that could explain the behavior of the subject in this event, described at the beginning of the introduction.

At that time, the operational instruments available were the following: ultra violet-visible light spectrophotometer and thin layer chromatography. A qualitative determination was made, since the time required to present the accusation was about to expire, therefore there was not enough time to establish the conditions to standardize a method, to obtain an internal standard that could achieve a certification. It should be noted that the cause of death was already determined, it was the consequence of a violent act and not by exogenous intoxication, due to an overdose of any psychoactive agent, drug of abuse or illicit substance.

The following are the characteristics that a standard or primary chemical standard must meet: Establishing a standard or standard of comparison is important, since it allows to evaluate the concentration or properties of another compound or analyte that must be identified, to provide answers to investigations that in the field of Forensic Medicine and Criminalistics are essential to clarify an alleged crime. For this purpose, an ideal primary chemical standard must comply with the following properties: 1) It must not react with or absorb the components of the atmosphere, such as water vapor, oxygen and carbon dioxide. 2) It should react according to an invariant reaction, 3) It should have a high degree of purity. 4) It must have a high molecular weight to minimize the effect of weighing error, 5) It must be soluble in the working solvent, 6) It must be non-toxic, 7) It must be readily available (cheap), 8) It must be environmentally friendly (Whitten, et al., 1998).

The following is a brief explanation of the aforementioned characteristics of a primary standard: a) Known chemical composition, which implies knowledge of its structure and elements that compose it, which will serve to perform the relevant stoichiometric calculations. b) High purity (98.5-99.9%), to avoid interferences, when performing the respective standardizations. c) Stable both at room temperature and at the temperature applied when dried in an oven (which is above the boiling point of water), thus avoiding errors in the measurements. d) It must not absorb gases or react with the components of the air, because this would lead to inaccuracies. e) It must react quickly and stoichiometrically with the standardizing agent, so that the calculations are as accurate as possible. f) High equivalent weight, which reduces measurement and weighing errors.

With reference to the analytical methods to be used in the research to be carried out, these are classified into classical and instrumental methods. The classical (definition), also called wet chemistry methods, preceded the instrumental methods by more than a century, the latter, although based on phenomena already certified more than a century ago, only managed to materialize with the development of electronics and computation (Skoog, et al., 2007).

This scientific basis will be used to support, by means of toxicological expertise, those cases where the ingestion of this alkaloid is presumed, and its link with any investigation on the violation of the Human Rights of Indigenous Peoples.

The exposition of diverse studies and methods carried out, will be the guide, to fulfill the requirements of a primary standard, and as a consequence to obtain a suitable internal standard for our analysis. In addition, the substance Supramencionada, is not very common in the routine of a forensic laboratory.

It is convenient to specify that chapter III or methodological framework indicates the type and design of the research that was developed, as well as the population, the sample used, in addition to the techniques and instruments that were used to collect the necessary data for the development of the research. Likewise, the results obtained are presented, as well as their analysis, and finally, the conclusions and recommendations obtained during the course of the research are specified.

forensic toxicology

Forensic Toxicology is the application of Toxicology for legal purposes (Poklis. 2005), that is, where there is a judicial investigation or presumption of malice, due to the use of a toxic agent to the detriment of a third party, thus providing elements of conviction, which will be useful both to the Administrators of Justice (Courts, Public Prosecutor's Office, Public Defender's Office) and to the criminal investigation agencies. This branch of Toxicology, related to Forensic Medicine and Criminalistics, will use and rely on state-of-the-art knowledge and technologies, which will allow a satisfactory response to the requirements of the aforementioned entities.

Establishing a standard or standard of comparison is important, since it allows to evaluate the concentration or properties of another compound or analyte that must be identified, to give answers to investigations that in the field of Forensic Medicine and Criminalistics are fundamental to clarify a presumed punishable act. For this, an ideal primary chemical standard must comply with the following properties: **1) It must not react**

with, nor absorb the components of the atmosphere, such as water vapor, oxygen and carbon dioxide. 2) It should react in accordance with an invariant reaction, 3) It should have a high degree of purity. 4) It must have a high molecular weight to minimize the effect of weighing error, 5) It must be soluble, 8) It must be harmless to the working solvent, 6) It must be non-toxic, 7) It must be readily available (cheap) to the environment (Whitten, et al., 1998).

The following is a brief explanation of the aforementioned characteristics that a primary chemical standard must meet: a) Known chemical composition, which implies knowledge of its structure and elements that compose it, which will serve to perform the relevant stoichiometric calculations. b) High purity (98.5-99.9%), to avoid interferences, when performing the respective standardizations. c) Stable both at room temperature and at the temperature applied when dried in an oven (which is above the boiling point of water), thus avoiding errors in the measurements. d) It should not absorb gases or react with air components, because this would lead to inaccuracies. e) It must react quickly and stoichiometrically with the standardizing agent, so that the calculations are as accurate as possible. f) High equivalent weight, which reduces measurement and weighing errors.

Forensic Toxicology, like other sciences, scientific or experimental disciplines, necessarily needs elements or patterns of comparison, which will indicate that the chemical-toxicological analysis, as well as the analytical steps used are adequate, since the toxic agent (analyte) obtained, visualized, measured, quantified at the end of the process, if it is the desired one, when compared, its characteristics must coincide with the agent already known and certified. Therefore it will be reported as a positive result, in the case of no match, the report will be negative, which will guarantee the suitability and certainty of the test performed.

For this purpose, analytical methods have been used with equipment and instruments such as ultraviolet-visible light spectrophotometer, separation techniques such as thin layer chromatography, among others, which allow determining in an exact and precise way the nature, composition, properties and qualities of a problem substance, within controllable variables and environments, which in addition to clarifying unknowns, relate it to a particular event in the criminalistic field and that merit both a scientific and legal investigation.

With reference to the above, analytical methods are classified into classical and instrumental. Classical methods **are called instrumental methods because they are the traditional methods of the late eighteenth century, the basic methods that every chemist should know, based on the chemical properties of the analyte, among these we have gravimetry, volumetry, among others.** It is worth mentioning that they also receive the name of wet chemistry methods, which preceded instrumental methods by more than a century, the **latter**, although based on phenomena already certified more than a century ago (last quarter of the nineteenth century), are based on the physicochemical properties of substances, among which are known spectroscopic, electroanalytical, thermal methods, among others, which only managed to materialize with the development of electronics and computation.(Skoog, and Cols, 2007).

Classical methods:

It should be added that in the early days of chemistry, most analyses were performed by separating the components of interest, the analytes, found in a sample by precipitation, extraction or distillation. In the case of qualitative analysis, the separated components were then treated with reagents that produced products, which could be identified by their color, boiling or melting temperatures, their solubilities in a range of solvents, their solubilities in a range of solvents, their odors, their optical activities or by their refractive indices. In the case of quantitative analysis, the amount of analyte was determined by gravimetric or volumetric measurements (Skoog et al., 2007).

In fact, gravimetric measurements determine the mass of the analyte or of some compound produced from it. In volumetric or titrimetric procedures, the volume or mass of a standard reagent needed to react with the analyte is measured. It should be noted that these classical methods for separating and determining analytes are still used in many laboratories. However, the extent of their general application is decreasing with the passage of time and with the emergence of instrumental methods to replace them (Skoog, et al., 2007).

Instrumental methods:

At the beginning of the 20th century, scientists began to exploit phenomena other than those used in classical methods to solve analytical methods. Thus, the measurement of physical properties of the analyte, such as conductivity, electrode potential, light absorption, mass-to-charge ratio and fluorescence began to be implemented in quantitative analysis. In addition, highly effective chromatographic and electrophoretic techniques began to replace distillation, extraction and precipitation as methods of separating components in complex mixtures prior to their qualitative or quantitative determination. These technological innovations, applied to separate and determine chemical species, are called *instrumental methods of analysis* (Skoog et al., 2007).

Probable dates for the introduction of the application of instrumental methods are shown below (Arango Gabriel "Alkaloids and Nitrogenous Compounds, 2008).

Date Instrumental method

1800 ------------------------------- Wet chemistry.

1950 Ultraviolet and infrared spectroscopy.

1960 Mass spectrometry, 1H NMR (60 - 100 MHz), Circular Dichroism.

1970 Carbon 13 --- nuclear magnetic resonance spectroscopy, high-field EM.

1980 ------------------ High resolution   NMR   (300-600   MHz),   correlations   and   two-dimensional techniques, computer aided.

   1990 Coupling techniques Chromatography (CPG, HPLC) -SM, NMR.

Now, these methods have allowed advances in the knowledge of the chemical properties of many botanical species for biomedical purposes, but also to understand the effects of the ingestion of plants in communities, particularly for ritual purposes. Regarding our American continent in its southern region and in particular the native peoples of the Amazonian area and El Chaco, the use of psychoactive substances for magical-therapeutic purposes extracted from plants, among which are mentioned ayahuasca, cebil, yopo (the subject of our study). A critical question is raised from the point of view of anthropology on the disparity of interpretations concerning the psychoactive capacity of these plant species. Taking as reference the work published by Linch (2008), where the social significance of cebil in the Wichi shamanism of the Chaco Salteno (geographical area between Argentina, Bolivia and Paraguay) is shown.

The testimony of the aborigines of that area, indicates that they process the seeds of the tree called by them Jataj (cebil), and the product obtained, they ingest it in their ceremonies, to achieve that spiritual journey, where they contact with the spirits, who eventually guide the shaman in their ancestral rituals. Western science classifies the cebil as genus Anadenanthera, species Columbrina, the effect of the active triptaminic principles of the cebil are qualified as hallucinogenic, that is to say, distorting the perception of reality.

It is appropriate to highlight the contribution of Valera (2015) regarding the shamanic healing of the Piaroa in the light of cultural heritage: the Piaroa are an Amerindian group of the Amazonas state, where special attention is paid to the processes of adaptation and cultural control exercised by this community, which preserves this ancestral practice and is complemented by health care from Western biomedicine. The socio-cultural implications within the community, the use of plants with their multiple effects, such as yopo (*Anadenanthera peregrina*), the significance of trance, communication with the spirits, the need for disease prevention, the maintenance of physical and spiritual health (traditional therapy), in coexistence with western medicine and health (Valera, 2015).

From the previous statements, it is concluded that the indigenous communities use botanical species such as the seeds of the yopo tree (as it is called by the indigenous communities and peoples of the Amazonas state, such as piaroa and yanomami) for ancestral magic-therapeutic practices. And that the optics of the western culture does not qualify it as a simple consumption of hallucinogenic substances and disrespecting their beliefs and cultural heritage.

On the other hand, two biological samples of human origin, of different nature (hematic and gastric), extracted from a corpse, which in life was presumed to have consumed the substance previously mentioned, were available. Each sample provides information on the pharmacology and toxicology of the compound, the route of administration and quantity taken, as well as the phenomena occurring after death. The interpretation of the results obtained remains the most important challenge for the forensic toxicologist (Soria et al., 2014), which allows to evaluate the suitability of each of them in terms of diagnosis, considering the ways of ingestion, pharmacokinetics and pharmacodynamics.

It should be said that blood is mainly a specialized transport medium (nutrients, oxygen, toxins, among others), of almost any substance or agent that enters the system of a living subject, therefore, what is found in it indicates consumption, absorption, which generates a response at the organic level, while what is found in the stomach and its contents indicates that it is the amount not absorbed, although it shows that it was ingested.

With reference to the above, Soria et al, 2014, state that the information provided by each sample and the interpretative difficulties arising as a result of a postmortem situation, the interest of these can be prioritized for chemico-toxicological studies as follows: Priority 1: blood, urine, vitreous humor and gastric content samples. Priority 2: bile, spleen, liver and kidney samples. Priority 3: brain, lung, hair and pericardial fluid samples. This means that blood is essential in all cases for the analysis of identification and quantification of the compounds to be investigated. Urine will provide information on the type of consumption by identifying the metabolites of interest, the vitreous humor is a representative matrix for qualitative analysis and the gastric content of a recent consumption.

Having made the above considerations, it is concluded that the importance of the rest of the evidences depends on their availability and the information they provide, which will depend on the limitation of the existing data in terms of toxicity and lethality, as well as on the correlations with the blood sample.

Therefore, samples classified as *priority 1* will always be the first choice and the others will be used when circumstances and maximum experience indicate it (etiology of death and type of toxic agent suspected).

RESEARCH BACKGROUND

In Venezuela we have as references about yopo studies and its effects, those made by Walter Coppens - Jorge Cato-David, published in Antropológica 28, 1971:3-24, which is entitled: "ASPECTOS ETNOGRAFICOS Y FARMACOLÓGICOS. THE YOPO AMONG THE CUIVA-GUAJIBO". As well as the one carried out by Granier-Doyeux, year 1948 and reflected in the Gaceta Médica de Caracas, 56,13-18, pag161-175, entitled: Acerca de una toxicomania indigena: el uso de la *Piptadenia peregrina* (nopo y y yopo).

In the work carried out by Coppens - Cato, they visited and observed the indigenous population cuiva - guajibo, established in San Esteban de Capanaparo, Apure State, in two periods. November 1969 and May 1970, collecting samples of the plant known as yopo, identified as *piptadenia peregrina* and classified as *Anadenanthera peregrina* (Shultes 1967:293).

The anthropologist dedicated himself to documenting the preparation of this alkaloid, as well as the frequency and symptoms caused by this hallucinogen, which is part of the ancestral customs and traditions of our indigenous peoples. They also marked the beginning of pharmacological studies to observe the effects of this toxic substance on laboratory animals (rats, mice, cats, dogs). Based on the data provided by Granier-Doyeux in 1948. The following tests were carried out:

1 Acute and chronic electroencephalographic studies in the cat, by means of the implantation of electrodes in different areas of the Central Nervous System.

2 .-) Recording of motor activity in mice, by means of a photoelectric cell actimeter.

3) Recording of blood pressure, heart rate, peripheral resistance and respiration in the dog.

4 .-) Recording of smooth muscle activity (nictitinous membrane) in the cat.

5 .-) Recording of the activity on the isolated rat uterus.

6 .-) Lethal dose 50 (LD50) and Lethal dose 95 (LD95) in mice.

The results obtained by Coppens were shown to be compatible with those of Granier-Doyeux. These were corroborated by Holmstedt and Lindgren (1967), who by applying gas chromatography (GC) and gas chromatography coupled to mass spectrometer (GC-MS), were able to separate from the seeds of *Piptadenia peregrina,* several active principles, identified as a series of substituted beta-phenethylamines: N,N- Dimethyltryptamine (DMT); N-Monomethyltryptamine (MMT); 5-Methoxy-N-N-N-Dimethyltryptamine (5-MeO-DMT); 5-Methoxy-N-Monomethyltryptamine (5-MeO-MMT); 5- Hydroxy-N-N-N-Dimethyltryptamine (5-OH-DMT, Bufotenine), of which DMT and 5-MeO-DMT were found to be potent psychotomimetic agents.

The results of this study were as follows:

1) They determined that yopo, pharmacologically, is a psychodysleptic, adrenergic hallucinogenic type, which according to its electroencephalographic record, behaves like LSD (lysergic acid diethylamide) and psilocybin type indolic derivatives, but less potent than these.

2 They concluded that the consumption of yopo among the cuiva-guajibo is mainly to establish relationships between individuals and families, who act as independent social units. They also observed a consumption that did not fulfill this role of link between different communities, but to evade the reality of the extermination of this community by Creole landowners.

Other researchers have made important contributions on the effects of N-N, Dimethyltryptamine (active principle of yopo), such as the one carried out by the American psychiatrist Rick Strassman, who monitored the effects of this hallucinogen in people who voluntarily volunteered for this experiment. Strassman mentions in his work entitled: **DMT: The spirit Molecule (DMT:**

The spirit Molecule, 2001), in the chapter entitled: **What is DMT,** the following: "that from the mid-1800s, explorers of the Amazon, in particular Richard Spruce of England and Alexander von Humboldt of Germany, described the effects of exotic cigarettes and beers made from plants by indigenous tribes. In the 20th century, the American botanist Richard Schultes continued this dangerous but exciting line of field work. Especially striking were the effects and the way of administering the rapépsicoactives ".

In the same chapter, he notes the following: "The indigenous tribes of Latin America continue to use these snuffs and have given them many names, such as yopo, epena and jurema. They take large doses, sometimes an ounce or more. A dramatic technique is for the inhalation partner to explode the powdered mixtures with considerable force through a tube or pipe into the other's nose. The energy of the explosion may be enough to drop the recipient to the ground.

He continues with the observations of Spruce and von Humboldt, who reported: "the natives were immediately incapacitated by these psychodelic strokes. Neither of the two, however, got to see for themselves what they were like. It was enough to see the Indians intoxicated, twitching, vomiting and babbling incoherently. These early explorers heard stories of fantastic visions, "out-of-body travel," predictions of the future, location of lost objects and contact with dead ancestors or other disembodied entities."

Following Spruce and von Humboldt's expedition, they took samples of these psychedelic plants from the New World to Europe. There the plants remained undisturbed for decades, as neither the interest nor the technology existed for a more detailed analysis of their chemical composition or their effects: "Another mixture of plants, consumed as a beverage, seemed to produce similar effects at a slower rate. This concoction also received several names, including ayahuasca and yage. This drink inspired much cave art and paintings drawn on the walls of native shelters, what today would be called "psychedelic" art.

Strassman states: "While psychedelic plants languished in the archives of the natural history museum, Canadian chemist R. Manske, in unrelated research, synthesized a new drug called N, N-dimethyltryptamine or DMT. As described in a 1931 scientific paper, Manske had manufactured several derivative compounds by chemically modifying tryptamine. He was interested in these products because they occurred in a toxic North American plant, the strawberry bush. DMT was one of these.

As far as is known, Manske made DMT, noted its structure and then placed his supply in a secluded corner of his laboratory, where he quietly collected dust. No one yet knew about the existence of DMT in plants that alter perception of the environment, its psychedelic properties, or its presence in the human body. There was little interest in psychedelics in scientific circles until decades later, after World War II.

In the early 1950s, the discoveries of LSD and serotonin shook the solid foundations of Freudian psychiatry and laid the groundwork for the new world of neuroscience. Curiosity about psychedelic drugs was intense in the growing circle of scientists who called themselves "psychopharmacologists". Chemists began probing the barks, leaves and seeds of plants first described as psychedelics a hundred years earlier for their active ingredients. The tryptamine family was a logical place to focus, since both serotonin and LSD are tryptamines.

The following is a chronological outline of the studies on DMT after 1931, as discussed in this chapter by Strassman:

1946: O. Gocalves isolated DMT from a South American tree used in tobacco production.

1955: M.S. Fish, N.M. Johson and E.C. Horning described the presence of

DMT in another tree related to tobacco production.

1955: Stephen Szara, Hungarian chemist and psychiatrist, emigrated to the United States and continued his studies on DMT, initiated in his country of origin in 1950. He discovered and documented that DMT is inactive orally, something that was already known to the indigenous people of the Amazon basin.

Yopo

YOPO: *Anadenanthera peregrina (L.) Speg.*

Scientific name: *Anadenanthera peregrina* (L.) Speg. (Synonym: Piptadenia peregrina (L.) Benth).

Common names: yopo (Venezuelan), yupa, curripaco, dopa, lomo de caimân (Colombian).

Anadenanthera peregrina is a tree from three (3) to eighteen (18) meters high, with a trunk of twenty (20) to fifty (50) millimeters in diameter and an expanded crown. It is distributed in South America (Colombia, to Brazil, Paraguay and Bolivia) and the Caribbean (Puerto Rico, Trinidad and Tobago), from sea level to 1100 meters elevation (1470 meters in Peru). It grows in the open plains of the plains of the Orinoco basin in Colombia and Venezuela, as well as in savannahs and open forests south of the Guianas. Yopal, the name of the capital of the Department of Casanare (Colombia), means place of yopos. In the West Indies, it has adapted, where it grows in open areas, low hills and poor soils, along watercourses (Vargas et al., 2013).

The bark of the yopo tree is thin, corky, rough, brown or gray. The leaves, 12 to 30 centimeters long, are bipinnate and have 10 to 40 leaflets. The inflorescences are formed by 35 to 50 small white flowers arranged in clusters. The fruit is a ribbon-shaped pod 1 to 5 centimeters long. The seeds are flattened yellowish brown and have a diameter of 1 to 3 millimeters, (Calle et al 2012), these seeds are easy and fast germination. The yopo plant is also used as a scattered tree in pastures, cultivated in lines in silvopastoral and agroforestry systems, as an ornamental species and for watershed protection (Calle et al. 2012) (Taken from Vargas et al., 2013).

Chemical properties

As already mentioned, the active principle obtained from the seeds of the yopo tree is *dimethyltryptamine (DMT),* hallucinogenic alkaloid, entheogenic *(magic-therapeutic context),* whose chemical name is *N,N-Dimethyl-1H-indole-3-ethanamine, chemical formula C12 H16 N2, molecular weight: 188.3. It is soluble in dilute acetic acid and in dilute mineral acids. Dimethyltryptamine (DMT),* can be presented in salt form, called *Dimethyltryptamine hydrochloride,* which is a white crystalline powder, with a melting point between 165° and 168°C. It is soluble in water. It should be added that its dissociation constant is 8.7 *(ethanol-water),* with a partition coefficient of 1.9 (octanol-water). When in contact with Marquis' Reagent (sulfuric acid with drops of formaldehyde), an orange coloration (color test) is obtained, indicating the possible presence of DMT.

It should be added that the separation method called Thin Layer Chromatography (TLC) can be used to extract it if DMT is part of a mixture, through the application of a simple technique. To reinforce the veracity of the result obtained with the TLC, the DMT is placed in an instrumental equipment called ultraviolet-visible light spectrometer, which should give readings for DMT of 279 nanometers (nm) in acidified aqueous solution and 288 (nm).

Alkaloids can be considered as: "An organic compound of natural origin (generally vegetable), nitrogenous (nitrogen is generally intracyclic), generally derived from amino acids, of more or less basic character, of restricted distribution, with important pharmacological properties at low doses and which respond to common precipitation reactions".

As for their natural state, alkaloids are essentially substances present in all organs of the plant, they can be found mainly in leaves (cocaine, nicotine, pilocarpine), flowers (scopolamine, atropine), fruits (opium alkaloids, peletiarine, coniine), seeds (piperine, arecoline), bark (quinine, tubocurarine), root (emetine and cephaline).

ROLE OF ALKALOIDS IN PLANTS

The function of alkaloids in plants is not yet clear, there are some suggestions about the "role" these substances play in plants such as:

• They serve as waste products or storage of excess nitrogen, this function is equivalent to that of uric acid or urea in animals.

• Since most alkaloids are associated with organic acids that facilitate their transport in the plant, they can serve as storage products for unmetabolized nitrogen or for nitrogen transport; in the case of the midritic Solanaceae, tropane esters are formed in the roots and transported to the aerial parts where they can be hydrolyzed.

• Microchemistry has shown in general that alkaloids are located in the peripheral tissues of the different organs of the plant, i.e. in the seed coat, stem bark, root or fruit and in the epidermis of the leaf; this allows us to think that alkaloids have an important function such as protecting the plant from insect attacks due to their bitter taste.

• Alkaloids can serve as growth regulators, it has been shown that putrescine-derived alkaloids increase markedly during germination of some plants such as barley, when they are found in potassium-deficient soils.

• Using biotechnological techniques, plants that normally accumulate alkaloids in the aerial parts, such as *Nicotiana* and *Daturas*, have been produced without alkaloids, the loss of alkaloids in the stem does not prevent the development of the plant, suggesting that alkaloids are not essential for plants.

Although the presence of alkaloids is not vital for the plant, they must participate in metabolic sequences and are not only waste products of metabolism (Arango Gabriel "Alkaloids and Nitrogenous Compounds, 2008).

ALKALOIDS DERIVED FROM TRYPTOPHAN (INDOLE ALKALOIDS)

The amino acid L-tryptophan contains the indole group and has its origin via the shikimic or anthranilic acid pathway.

From the pharmacological point of view, there is much interest in the bases containing the indole nucleus, following the discovery of the hallucinogenic activity of LSD as well as the sedative activity of reserpine, isolated from the genus *Rauwolfia*, the peak of this phytochemical study occurred in the 60's and was mainly directed to the Apocynaceae family.

There are about 800 alkaloids of this type distributed mainly in the Apocynaceae family (genera *Rauwolfia*, *Aspidos-perma*, *Strychnos* and *Vinca*), less frequent in fungi and families such as Leguminoseae, Malphigiaceae, Rubiaceae and Rutaceae where the alkaloids present the simple indole group.

Tryptophan is the precursor of these alkaloids, which are classified into tryptamines and non-tryptamines; tryptamines, in turn, are subdivided into β-carbolines and indolenines and can be simple tryptamines or complex tryptamines and these can be isoprenic or non-isoprenic.

SINGLE TRYPTAMINES

Simple tryptamines play an important role in the indigenous culture of the Americas for their hallucinogenic and ecstatic effects in their magical-religious ceremonies; They have been found in Mesoamerican hallucinogenic mushrooms of the genera *Psilocybe, Stropharia* and *conocybe* ("teonacatl" or "flesh of the gods") used by the Aztec Indians in their religious ceremonies for more than 1700 years. The hallucinogenic alkaloids psilocybin and psilibin have been found in these mushrooms, which when ingested produce different auditory and visual sensations, muscular relaxation, depressions and alternating euphoria. Serotonin, which plays an important role in neuronal activity, is also found in vegetables and has been isolated in the pericarp of the banana, which, when smoked when dried, acts as a mild hallucinogen.

Simple tryptamines by decarboxylation, methylation and oxidation reactions of tryptophan.

From the parotid glands of the common toad *Bufo vulgaris* is isolated the N-dimethylated derivative bufotenin of serotonin which is also the active principle of Yopo, powder from the seeds of *Anadenanthera peregrina (Piptadenia peregrina)* Leguminoseae and species of the genus *Virola* (Myristicaceae), are mixed with ashes and inhaled through bamboo tubes by the Orinoco Indians in magic-religious ceremonies producing hallucination and motor incoordination.

Among the simple tryptamines are included slightly more complex structures such as ergine, an alkaloid extracted from the Convulvulaceae of the New World considered sacred plants of Mexico called "snake plant" have been used in the Aztec empire by shamans in magical religious ceremonies to know the future, cure diseases or in religious sacrifices; physostigmine or eserin and eseroline found in *Physostigma venenosum* (Leguminoceae), a Guinea vine that produces a large pod with 2 or 3 seeds 2 to 3 cm long known as calabar beans, used in Africa in ordeals as oral hallucinogens, their ingestion produces hypersecretion: saliva, sweat, tears and urine, visual disturbances, thirst, trembling, contractions and sometimes death by cardiac arrest.

Yagé, ayahuasca or caapi is the bark of the liana of the genus *Banisteriopsis* Family Malpighiaceae of the Amazon and Orinoquia, found mainly in *B. caapi, B.inebrians and B. rusbiana* where bases such as harmala and harmaline have been extracted, the latter used in the treatment of Parkinson's disease.

Alkaloids of this type were also found in *Pegamun harmala* (Zygophillaceae) and in lesser quantities in families Rutaceae, Leguminoceae, Rubiaceae and Passifloraceae in the genus *Passiflora*. The ingestion of yagé produces hallucinogenic and divinatory effects in shamans.

There is a type of alkaloid which has an indole nucleus with a single nitrogen in its structure, of the carbazole type isolated from the Rutaceae family, specifically from the genus *Muraya*, this type of alkaloids have also been isolated as dimers with important cytotoxic activity.

Traditionally, the species of the genus *Muraya* have been used for analgesia and local anesthesia, treatment of eczema, rheumatism, abdominal pain, hydropesia, diarrhea, edema, thrombosis, venous ecstasy, anticonvulsant and expectorant; from the chemical point of view it has been found that this genus presents flavonoid coumarins, carbazole type alkaloids (Arango Gabriel "Alkaloids and Nitrogenous Compounds, 2008).

Dimethyltryptamine

Dimethyltryptamine (DMT), inactivated when ingested orally, is rapidly metabolized after intramuscular administration and almost entirely transformed first into indole-3-ylacetic acid. About 33% of a dose is excreted in the urine after 6 hours in free form and as a conjugate (glucuronic) in *indole-3-ylacetic acid, less than 0.1% of the dose is excreted unchanged in the urine within 24 hours. On the other hand,* the concentration of endogenous DMT is less than 0.001mg/L. 15 male volunteers, aged 26 to 48 years, were administered 2 ml/kg of *hoasca tea, a sacred Amazonian brew, whose alkaloid content was as follows: DMT = 0.24mg/ml; harmine =1.70mg/ml; harmaline = 0.20mg/ml; tetrahydroharmine= 1.07mg/ml.* The peak plasma concentration was 15.8 micrograms per liter, after 107.5 minutes coinciding with the peaks of psychoactivity (J.C. Callaway et al., J Ethnofharmacol., 1999, 65,243-256). Clarke's anus, 2005.

Shamanic Ritual Use of Yopo in Venezuela

To address the use of yopo by indigenous population groups in Venezuelan territory, as a shamanic ritual, it is convenient to address the contribution of research conducted by Valera Emanuel and published in 2015, where he refers to the following: "Shamanism constitutes a set of beliefs, practices and traditional rituals that are oriented to the diagnosis and healing of the suffering that the human being presents, this through the contact of the shaman with the world of the spirits, constituting a sort of intermediary between the natural world and the higher world, this institution involves a group of people with specialized knowledge unlike what happens in animism where everyone practices it".

He also refers that: "The basis of shamanism is based on the coexistence of different dimensions, where a visible world is affected by non-visible spiritual forces and entities that are located in parallel realities of simultaneous temporality". Coinciding and quoting Mircea Eliade (1964), he reaffirms: "shamans are found in various parts of the world, and their main characteristic is that they act as doctors and spiritual guides, this through their communication with the world of the spirits, from techniques that induce trance which incites the ecstasy of visions, seeking answers for the resolution of problems in the community or village where they reside, especially those related to health".

Valera, agrees with other scholars on the use of the term shaman, for the designation of the intermediary operator, magician, sorcerer, or healer, depending on the socio-cultural constitution of the society where it is found, and its origin, and for this he cites the most important authors such as: "Eliade with his position of the characterization of shamanism, Kehoe with his criticism towards what was disseminated by the latter, by virtue of the fact that he had not carried out work with direct observation of the practices to which he refers and Hoppàl with the proposal of the use of the term "shamanism" as a possibility of marking the variability and specificity in local cultures, for the purposes of this research work it has been agreed to use the adjective "shamanism", as the derivation of the practices exercised by a healer who communicates with the world of the spirits".

As Llamazares (2013, p.69) points out "one of the fundamental themes of shamanic knowledge is related to the ability to heal both physical illnesses and spiritual disorders", so that it constitutes an integrative and multidimensional vision of what is conceived as reality, of the individual and the phenomenon of health-disease, being its therapeutic quality that healing potential coupled with a spiritual power, however, in contemporary times it has certainly undergone changes, as culture is dynamic.

In this approach we try to analyze the phenomenon of shamanic healing from the perspectives and terms of the Piaroa culture, an Amerindian population group that resides in the states of Amazonas and Bolivar, in the extreme west of the Guiana Shield of the Bolivarian Republic of Venezuela, occupying different territorial spaces of the humid jungle, These include river basins such as the Sipapo, Cuao, Marieta, Cataniapo and Samariapo, among others, but they have also settled along the northern and southern road axes of Puerto Ayacucho, as well as in the department of Vichada in Colombia (Bello, 2010).

In this sense, the analysis will focus on the scientific literature written so far on this topic and the field work carried out by the author in the period between 2008 and 2011 in the Piaroa community of Alto Carinagua, in the municipality of Atures, Amazonas state, in collaboration with the Student Research Group for Social Sciences (GIECS) of the Central University of Venezuela.

It presents a description of the processes involved in the path to becoming a shaman, the scope of the practice, the ritual events that sustain shamanic healing, the socio-cultural implications within the community, the use of plants with their multiple effects, the significance of trance and communication with spirits, the need for disease prevention and maintenance of physical and spiritual health, as well as traditional therapeutics.

Likewise, we explore the relationships generated by the welfare intervention from the western biomedical health apparatus and shamanic healing in this community, as elements related to the cultural control exercised by the Piaroa inhabitants of the aforementioned area, operate for the preservation and coexistence of their traditional healing practices with respect to the use of medicines from the pharmaceutical industry and the syncretism that is produced in the therapy in certain cases.

Now, it is important to consider when speaking of Piaroa shamanism, what Lévi-Strauss (1958) exposed, by virtue of the symbolic efficacy, since there is a correspondence between the terms of the mythological story and the anatomical and physiological structure of the individual who suffers, in the case of the author with respect to what he points out about the difficult births among the Cuna Indians and the role of the shaman, in the case of the Piaroas with respect not only to this type of events but also to the general configuration of the phenomenon of health and illness.

As Lévi-Strauss (1958, p. 173) indicates, "the shaman does not touch the body of the sick person and does not administer a remedy. 173) indicates "the shaman does not touch the body of the sick person and does not administer a remedy; but, at the same time, he directly and explicitly discusses the pathological state and its localization: we would gladly say that the chant constitutes a "psychological manipulation" of the sick organ and that from this manipulation the cure is expected", in the same way in the piaroa shamanic healing, there is no direct contact with the organs, if the sick person refers headache, the shaman uses a ritual maraca and passes it around the head and with the mouth sucks without contact, the cause of the ailment and then spits it to the side.

This symbolic efficacy is therefore understood as healing since the person suffering from the disease in his process of understanding "(...) does more than resign himself: he is cured" (Lévi-Strauss, 1958, p. 178), since the fact is given, "(...) the symbols of the myth, summoned in the ritual process, manage to unblock the physiological process" (Gonzàlez, 2009, p. 9).

Precisely, as it will be observed in the development of the text, the preservation of this tradition among the Piaroas, gives account of this symbolic effectiveness, and it is constituted as a mechanism for the transmission of this knowledge to the following generations, being therefore an intergenerational inheritance, where several elements are structured in the same institution, which allows social cohesion.

Thus, from a patrimonial perspective, historical consciousness, which Arregui (1988, p. 182) points out on the basis of Dilthey's conception, "(.) is not only to know that there is a past, and that this past conditions the present, but rather to notice the irreducible plurality of situations and states of life. To become aware of history is to become aware of human diversity" and it is precisely in this sense that this awareness, sustained by symbolic efficacy, is erected as the mechanism for the legitimization of practices, and which is simultaneously transmitted through time by orality and the use of shamanic therapy, tradition is not a fact of the past, but constitutes an indivisible and intertemporal bridge between ancestral knowledge and the present, as it represents part of the cultural ethos of that people and the ways of facing situations in the process of health and illness.

Indigenous communities and peoples that use it

Among the indigenous populations that use the yopo we have: The Cuiva, who linguistically belong to the Guajibo group, which are concentrated in Venezuela in the Llanos, in two populations, both located along the Capanaparo river. The total population of the Cuiva still surviving in Venezuela at the time of Coppen's research, after repeated genocides perpetrated against this group, probably did not reach 400 individuals.

Other Cuiva-speaking groups, or those speaking very similar dialects, live scattered in the plains of Venezuela and Colombia, concentrated mainly in the regions of the Arauca, Cinaruco, Meta and Casanare rivers.

Another indigenous population that uses this hallucinogenic alkaloid are the Piaroa, and citing the work of Valera, 2015."The aim is to analyze the phenomenon of shamanic healing from the perspectives and terms of the Piaroa culture, an Amerindian population group that resides in the states of Amazonas and Bolivar, in the western end of the Guiana Shield of the Bolivarian Republic of Venezuela, occupying different territorial spaces of the rainforest, which include river basins such as the Sipapo, Cuao, Marieta, Cataniapo and Samariapo, among others, but they have also settled in the northern and southern road axes of Puerto Ayacucho, also in the department of Vichada, in the Colombian territory there are also Piaroa settlements (Bello, 2010)".

Valera conducted her fieldwork between 2008 and 2011 in the Piaroa community of Alto Carinagua, in the municipality of Atures, Amazonas state, in collaboration with the Student Research Group for Social Sciences (GIECS) of the Central University of Venezuela.

In this research, the above-mentioned researcher details the process to be followed for an individual of this community to become a shaman, the scope of the practice, the ritual events that sustain shamanic healing, the socio-cultural implications within the community, as well as: "the use of plants with their multiple effects, the significance of trance and communication with the spirits, the need for disease prevention and maintenance of physical and spiritual health, as well as traditional therapeutics".

Ways of preparation

The Cuiva people collect yopo during its flowering season, which goes from December to April, yopo occupies a preponderant position in the daily life of the Cuiva. At almost any time of the day, an indigenous person can be observed in the process of opening yopo pods or absorbing the hallucinogenic powder. Women are frequently incorporated in the task of extracting yopo seeds; but only a few participate in the actual consumption. Women also take part in the collection of the pods. After collecting the seeds, the Cuiva leaves them to dry for several days in a sunny place. At the end of drying, the Indian compresses the vegetable mass and then applies it to the outer wall of a mortar that is normally used to crush the various types of tubers that enter into the Cuiva diet. Now he begins to crush the mass with a small stick, until it is completely soft.

The only non-vegetable substance that goes into the preparation of yopo is the snail shell (WARURO). After having reduced the shell in several small pieces, the Indian places them in a brazier, until they reach the point of incandescence. The snail pieces, which have now taken on a white color, are then placed on a wooden tray.

The palette (PATE), which is used to grind the various substances that finally compose the yopo, comes from a single piece of wood. The Cuiva; carves this wood with machete and knife; the polishing of the surface of the paddle is done with rough blades.

With a hand (NATUTO) the Indian begins to gradually reduce the pieces of shell into a very fine powder. At the end of this operation, the powder thus obtained is mixed with the yopo mass that has been detached from the wall of the mortar. If necessary, when the mass coming from the mixture of yopo and snail shell is not soft enough, it is necessary to re-apply the paste on the external wall of the mortar for the final softening sequence.

The next stage consists of placing the mixed yopo dough, in the manner of a small flat cake, on a fork-shaped stick (TANEBÜDÜ). The Indian places the tija over a small overwhelming fire. When the paste has reached a sufficient degree of consistency and the moisture has been completely absorbed, the Cuiva removes the tija from the fire.

Now the process that consists of reducing the mass of yopo mixed in powder can begin. The cake is placed in the palette previously described, the same one that has served to reduce the fragments of conch shell. The Cuiva crushes the dough with the hand until the paste is completely reduced. From this moment the yopo can be consumed.

Forms of ingestion

When the time has come to take the hallucinogen, the Cuiva pours the powder in a thin layer on the wooden palette, in doses that generally do not exceed 5 grams per intake. The yopo (DOPA) is

The Indian has an adapted absorbing instrument at his disposal for this purpose. The utensil (SIRUPO) consists of a hollow bone, to which are connected two heron bones in whose extremities appear perforated nuggets of palm. These extremities fit with the nostrils, through which the Cuiva deeply and vigorously inhales the hallucinogenic powder.

During the intake itself, we often observe that nasal and respiratory tract irritation is the cause of severe vomiting.

At the end of the intake of yapa, most individuals - even the older ones who have long been in the habit of consuming the hallucinogen - vomit repeatedly. Some Indians artificially provoke vomiting by inserting a finger or a bird feather in the mouth.

After having finished the absorption of the powder, many individuals present a black nasal stream dripping along the upper lip of the mouth. In addition, there are a number of other external symptoms: bulging eyes and widened pupils, with the gaze fixedly directed forward; sometimes the eyes appear bloodshot; facial or head twitching. Some of them have an abrupt access of exuberance and start singing (loudly).

The yopo also has the particularity to present them the surrounding things "more beautiful", more colorful, but with a predominance of a soft white color. They also added that yopo gives them a lot of strength to work and to dance.

In fact, after the first sequences, it often happens that the drugged person immediately goes out to work, with a great external display of energy. In other cases, the individual withdraws in his or her hammock, claiming to be very "drunk". The duration of the "recovery" sequence varies on average between a quarter of an hour and a maximum of two hours.

The symptomatology of yopo as it manifests itself among the Cuiva generally corresponds to other observations made on the consumption of *piptadenia pqregrina.* These observations, made basically in the Orinoco basin and adjacent zones, which is the area of distribution of the *legume* (COOPER 1949: 536-537), make a distinction as to the effects that the consumption of the hallucinogen can have. The first symptoms are described as stimulating, and are accompanied by visual hallucinations and a great motor activity of the subject. The later phase is characterized by a tendency of the individual to reduce his movements and to sleep (GRANIER-DOYEUX 1948: 168; SCHULTES 1969: 249).

One of the most obvious functions of collective consumption of yopo, as well as community dances, is to channel peaceful social interaction between individuals from families who, under normal circumstances, tend to act in complete autonomy from other family units, which means that they have rather limited mutual contacts.

DESCRIPTION OF THE SAMPLES ANALYZED, ANALYTICAL PROGRESS AND CONCLUSIONS.

a) A set of eleven (11) seeds of *Anadenanthera peregrina*, six of them from the *Yanomami* indigenous community of Alto Parima (Amazonas state) and five from the collection of the Caracas Botanical Garden, donated to this institution by the anthropologist América Perdomo of the Amazonian Center for Research and Control of Tropical Diseases (CAICET).

b) Biological samples of human origin, hematological (blood) and gastric (stomach contents).

To achieve the extraction of the active principle of concern in this case, the seeds from the plant called yopo *(Piptadenia / Anadenanthera peregrina)*, were subjected to a relevant analytical procedure, which will be described below:

Method for the extraction of DMT from yopo seeds.

1 Two (2) yopo seeds were taken and weighed.

2 .-) They were placed in a mortar to proceed to crushing them with a pestle or piloncillo, until pulverization.

3) The product of the finely divided seeds is taken up with 10 milliliters of distilled water or, failing that, with ethanol for analysis and poured into a separating funnel.

4 .-) It is alkalinized with (drops) of concentrated ammonium hydroxide until reaching a ph= 11.

5 .-) 20 milliliters of chloroform for analysis are added.

6 .-) It is shaken as indicated by the appropriate technique for the case.

7) We separate the chlorophoric layer, the volume obtained is measured.

8) Three portions, each one of 2 milliliters of the organic phase are taken, each one is poured in its respective porcelain capsule (one for chemical

reaction, one for chromatography in thin layer and another one for spectrophotometric reading).

9 .-) They are placed under a fume hood, until total evaporation.

10 .-) The pertinent determinations are made.

Methodology to be followed to work the biological samples and determine which psychoactive substance is found in them (both in organs and biological fluids).

1) The evidence to be analyzed is photographically fixed.

2 .-) Then the salient features of the evidence are described, in this particular case, it was done in the following way:

In fact, the biological fluid (blood) collected during the medico-legal autopsy on the body of the Yanomami Indian was processed to verify if the victim consumed any psychoactive substance that could explain the behavior of the subject in this event, as described at the beginning of the introduction.

At that time, the operational instruments available were the following: ultra violet-visible light spectrophotometer and thin layer chromatography. A qualitative determination was made, since the time required to present the accusation was about to expire, therefore there was not enough time to establish the conditions to standardize a method, to obtain an internal standard that could achieve a certification. It should be noted that the cause of death was already determined, it was the consequence of a violent act and not by exogenous intoxication, due to an overdose of any psychoactive agent, drug of abuse or illicit substance.

This case finally demonstrated the importance of having internal standards of chemical substances or agents in the Forensic Science Laboratories (UCCVDF-AMC), and in non-routine cases, when they are not available, to cultivate institutional relationships with other organizations related to our objectives and functions. In this opportunity we had the valuable collaboration of the Victor Manuel Ovalles Herbarium of the Faculty of Pharmacy of the Central University of Venezuela. As well as the wisdom of anthropologists attached to the UCCVDF-AMC, to settle everything related to the violation of fundamental rights, especially that of indigenous peoples.

RESULTS

SAMPLE RECEIVED	QUANTITY	PH	Ethyl Alcohol	RESULTS FOR ALKALOIDS
Gastric Content	30 ml	4	NEGATIVE	
Blood	30 ml		NEGATIVE	Dimethyltryptamine

Source: Author's acquis.

CONCLUSIONS

Based on the chemical and toxicological analysis of the studied evidences, which motivates the present expert action, it is concluded:

In the sample corresponding to the corresponding corpse, who in life responded to the name of **XXX.** Analyzed by chemical reactions, thin layer chromatography and UV spectrophotometry, **it was detected in the blood sample, the presence of Dimethyltryptamine, which is an alkaloid with hallucinogenic properties, obtained from the seed of the plants Anadenanthera Peregrina or Piptadenia Peregrina, commonly known in the region of the Amazonas state with the name of YOPO.**

REFERENCES

• VIRTUAL PORTALS

• Clarke's. Analysis Of Drugs And Poisons (2005) (November 26, 2013).

• Usda, Ars, National Genetic Resources Program. Germplasm Resources Information Network - (grin) [online database]. National Germplasm Resources Laboratory, Beltsville, Maryland. url: http://www.ars-grin.gov/cgi-

bin/npgs/html/gnlist.pl?1463 (November 26, 2013).

• BIBLIOGRAPHIC REFERENCES

• Arango Acosta, Gabriel Jaime. Alkaloids and Nitrogenous Compounds. University of Antioquia, Medellin, Colombia. June 2008).

• Coppens Walter, Cato-David Jorge. Ethnographic and Pharmacological Aspects "The Yopo among the Cuiva-Guajibo". Antropologia 28, 1971,3:24. Caracas. Venezuela.

• Garcia-Rodriguez S, Giménez Mp. 2005. Human and instrumental resources in a forensic toxicology laboratory. Revista De Toxicologia. Pp. 1-11.

• Lizot J. 2005. The Yanomami (Yanomami). In: Salud Indigena De Venezuela. Ministerio Del Poder Popular Para La Salud.

• Linch, Fernando. The Spirit of the Khatâj. A Perspectivist Reading Of The Psychoactivity Of The Cebil In Wichi Shamanism, 2008.

• Poklis, Alphonse. Chapter 31. Casarett and Doull, Fundamentos De Toxicologia. Klaassen, C. et al. Editorial. Mcgraw-Hill. Interamericana 2005.

• Repetto, M y Cols. Fundamental Toxicology, Fourth Edition, 2009. Diaz De Santos Editions.

• Strassman, Rick. The spirit of the molecule. Publisher: Park Street

Press. (2001).

• Soria Y Cols Interés De Las Muestras Para Los Estudios Quimico-Toxicológicos *Post Mortem* the Value Of Samples For Postmortem Toxicological Studies ,2014.

• Vargas Raùl, et al. Degree work to obtain the title of Forestry Engineer, 2013.

• Whitten, K et al, General Chemistry. Fifth Edition. Editorial McGraw-Hill. Interamericana de Espana.1998.

-

• **LEGAL REFERENCES**

• Law on Cultural Heritage of Indigenous Peoples and Communities. 2009.

• National Constitution of the Bolivarian Republic of Venezuela. 1999.

• Organic Law of Indigenous Peoples and Communities. 2012.

• Organic Law on Drugs. 2013.

• Organic Code of Criminal Procedure. 2012.

• Penal Code. 2012.

Glossary of basic terms and annexes

• **Absorption (biological): The** process of entry or transport, active or passive, of a substance into an organism; can take place through different pathways.

• **Administration (of a substance):** Application of a known quantity of a substance to an organism by a defined route and reproducible procedure.

• **Alkaloid:** is an organic compound of nitrogenous type produced by certain plants. These compounds generate **physiological effects** of different kinds, which are the basis of drugs such as cocaine and morphine.

• **Hallucinogen: Hallucinogens** are drugs that, in non-toxic doses, cause profound alterations in the user's perception of reality. Under their influence, people see images, hear things and experience sensations very different from those of wakefulness. Some hallucinogens also produce rapid and intense emotional oscillations. On the negative side, they often produce mental confusion, loss of memory or disorientation in space and time.

• **Anadenantera Peregrina:** is a perennial tree native to the Caribbean and South America.

• **Qualitative analysis:** is a branch of analytical chemistry that aims at the recognition or identification of the elements or chemical groups present in a sample, as well as the study of the means to identify the chemical components of a sample. In general, the basis for the identification of a substance by the classical method of analysis consists in provoking a change in its properties that is easily observable and that corresponds to the constitution of the substance.

• **Quantitative Analysis:** is the determination of the absolute/relative abundance (often expressed as concentration) of one, several or all of the chemical substances present in a sample. Once the presence of a certain substance in a sample is known, the quantification or measurement of its absolute or relative abundance can help in the determination of its specific properties.

- **Analyte:** is a component (element, compound or ion) of analytical interest in a sample that is separated by chromatography. It is a chemical species whose presence or content is to be known, identifiable and quantifiable, by means of a chemical measurement process.

- **Ayahuasca:** is a traditional indigenous drink of the Amazonian and Andean peoples of the tropical and subtropical areas of South America. The drink is a decoction with a long history of entheogenic use formed by mixing banisteriopsis caapi (yagé or ayahuasca), which contains harmine and tetrahydroharmine (THH), alkaloids of the beta-carboline class, which act as monoamine oxidase inhibitors (MAOI) and allow the primary psychoactive component Dimethyltryptamine (DMT) to become active; and a second plant that has the DMT itself, namely psychotria viridis, also known as *chacrona*; diplopterys cabrerana, known as *chagropanga* or *chaliponga*; brunfelsia splendida; brugmansia suaveolens, known as trompetero, floripondio, tomapende or toé; and banisteriopsis rubyana.

- **Shaman:** is the one who is attributed the ability to modify reality or the collective perception of it, in a way that does not respond to a causal logic. This can be finally expressed, for example, in the ability to heal, to communicate with the spirits and to present visionary and divinatory abilities. It is the term used to indicate this type of person, present mainly in the hunter-gatherer societies of Asia, Africa, America and Oceania and also in prehistoric cultures of Europe.

- **Forensic Sciences:** are a set of scientific disciplines that help police and justice to determine the exact circumstances of the commission of an offense and to identify its perpetrators.

- **Indigenous Communities:** These are human groups formed by indigenous families associated among themselves, belonging to one or more indigenous peoples, which are located in a given geographical area and organized according to the cultural patterns of each people, with or without modifications from other cultures.

• **Congeners:** Of the same genus, of the same origin or of the same derivation.

• **Thin Layer Chromatography:** is a chromatographic technique that uses a vertically immersed plate. This chromatographic plate consists of a polar stationary phase (usually silica gel) adhered to a solid surface. The stationary phase is a uniform layer of an absorbent held on a plate, which may be glass, aluminum or other support.

• **Cosmogony:** is any theoretical model that tries to explain the origin and development of the Universe. In astronomy, cosmogony studies the origin of certain astrophysical objects or systems, the Solar System or the Earth-Moon system. In the past, cosmogonic theories were part of different religions and mythologies. However, thanks to the evolution of science, it is now based on the study of various astronomical phenomena.

• **Dimethyl Tryptamine (DMT):** is an entheogen. It is found normally in nature, and pharmacologically belongs to the tryptamine family. Many cultures, indigenous and modern, ingest DMT as an entheogen, in extracts or in synthesized form.

• **Endocannibalism:** Practice, custom or rite of consuming human flesh by beings of the same species (also anthropophagy). The Yanomami practice a certain endocannibalism by consuming, in a ritual, the ashes of their dead.

• **Comparison Standard:** it is the norm in which a previously established comparison group is available, from which the standards or norms are defined to which the results obtained by each of the students in a course are compared, when a procedure is applied to detect the expected learning for a unit.

- **Stupefacient:** Substance that decreases the activity of the nervous system and, consequently, the psychic and mental activity. (see. Eng.) syn. Narcotic.

- **Spectrophotometer:** an instrument used in chemical analysis to measure, as a function of wavelength, the relationship between values of the same photometric quantity relative to two beams of radiation and the concentration or chemical reactions measured in a sample. It is also used in chemistry laboratories for the quantification of substances and microorganisms.

- **Drug:** In a broad sense, any product that can be absorbed by an organism, diffuse in it and produce changes in it, favorable or otherwise. Drugs used for the diagnosis and treatment of diseases are medicines. Syn.: xenobiotic.

- **Pharmacokinetics:** is the branch of pharmacology that studies the processes to which a drug is subjected during its passage through the body. It tries to elucidate what happens to a drug from the moment it is administered until its total elimination from the body.

- **Pharmacodynamics:** is the study of the biochemical and physiological effects of drugs and their mechanisms of action and the relationship between the concentration of the drug and its effect on an organism. In other words, it is the study of what happens to the organism by the action of a drug. From this point of view, it is the opposite of pharmacokinetics, which studies the processes to which a drug is subjected during its passage through the organism.

- **Guajibo (jivi): they** are an indigenous people living in the Orinoco Plains, between the Guaviare, Meta and Arauca rivers, in the Colombian departments of Vichada, Meta (Puerto Gaitân and Mapiripân), Arauca, Guaviare and Guainia, and in Venezuela to the west of the states of Amazonas, Bolivar and south of Apure.

- **Indigenous habitat:** The set of physical, chemical, biological and socio-cultural elements that constitute the environment in which indigenous peoples and communities develop and allow the development of their traditional ways of life. It includes the soil, water, air, flora, fauna and in general all those material and immaterial resources necessary to guarantee the life and development of indigenous peoples and communities.

- **Indigenous:** Any person descending from an indigenous people, who inhabits the geographic space and who maintains the cultural, social and economic identity of his people or community, recognizes himself as such and is recognized by his people and community, even if he adopts elements from other cultures.

- **Inhumation:** Burial of a corpse.

- **Intoxication:** Pathological process, with clinical signs and symptoms caused by a substance of exogenous or endogenous origin.

- **In vivo:** Study performed on a living individual. Ant. in vitro.

- **Forensic medicine:** also called forensic medicine, medical jurisprudence or judicial medicine, is the branch of medicine that applies all the medical and biological knowledge necessary for the resolution of the problems posed by the law. The forensic physician assists judges and courts in the administration of justice by determining the origin of injuries sustained by a wounded person or the cause of death by examining a corpse.

- **Traditional indigenous medicine:** Comprises the body of knowledge of biodiversity, as well as the practices, ideas, beliefs and procedures related to physical and mental illnesses or social imbalances of a given indigenous people and community. This body of knowledge explains the etiology and procedures for diagnosis, prognosis, healing, disease prevention and health promotion. It is transmitted by tradition from generation to generation within indigenous peoples and communities.

- **Gravimetric measurements:** consists of the measurement of the gravity field. It is usually used when the object of study is the gravity field or the density variations responsible for its variation.

- **Metabolite: A** substance that the body makes or uses when it breaks down food, drugs or chemicals; or its own tissue (e.g., fat or muscle tissue). This process, called metabolism, produces energy and materials needed for growth, reproduction and maintenance of health. It also helps to eliminate toxic substances.

- **Sample:** 1) Portion of material selected from a larger quantity so that the fraction chosen is representative of the whole. If possible, the whole should be homogenized before sampling. 2) In statistics: a group of individuals taken at random from a population for research purposes. 3) One or more specimens taken from a population or a process with the intention of obtaining information from them. T. rel. Random sample, random sample, stratified sample, systematic sample.

- **LSD: Lysergic acid diethylamide**, **LSD-25** or simply **LSD** (from the German *Lysergsaure-Diethylamid*), also called **lysergide** and commonly known as **acid**, is a semi-synthetic psychedelic drug derived from ergoline and the tryptamine family that produces psychological effects.

- **Equivalent Weight:** Also called combination weight is the amount of a substance capable of combining or displacing 1 part by mass of H2, 8 parts by mass of O2 or 35.5parts by mass of Cl2.

- **Piaroa:** indigenous people living on the banks of the Orinoco and its tributary rivers in present-day Venezuela and in some other areas of Venezuela and Colombia.

- **Traditional economic practices:** Traditional economic practices are considered to be those carried out by indigenous peoples and communities within their habitat and lands, in accordance with their needs and their own cultural patterns, which include their techniques and procedures for production, distribution and consumption of goods and services, their forms of cultivation, breeding, hunting, fishing, elaboration of products, use of natural resources and forest products for food, pharmacological purposes and as raw material for the manufacture of housing, boats, implements, utilitarian, ornamental and ritual implements, as well as their traditional forms and intra and inter-community exchange of goods and services. Innovation in economic practices in indigenous peoples and communities does not affect their traditional character.

•	**Psychedelic:** is a psychic state of a person who is under the influence of a hallucinogen. It causes the individual to have a perception of hitherto unknown aspects of the mind, and alters consciousness, bringing sensations similar to sleep, psychosis and religious ecstasy.

•	**Psilocybin:** (also known as **4-PO-DMT**) is an alkaloid prodrug of the classic hallucinogenic compound psilocin, responsible for the psychoactive effect of the drug. Both drugs are members of the indole and tryptamine classes of drugs.

•	**Indigenous Peoples:** Human groups descending from the original peoples that inhabit the geographic space corresponding to the national territory, who recognize themselves as such, by having one or some of the following elements: ethnic identities, lands, social, economic, political, cultural institutions, and their own justice systems, which distinguish them from other sectors of the national society and which they are determined to preserve, develop and transmit to future generations.

•	**Scott's reagent: also called cobalt thiocyanate test** is a chemical test proven to show the presence of cocaine. The cobalt thiocyanate reagent can be prepared by dissolving 10 g of cobalt (II) thiocyanate in a mixture of 490 mL of distilled water and 500 mL of glycerol.

•	**Marquis reagent:** form of a portable test, designed for the preliminary identification of alkaloids, narcotics, methamphetamines, analgesics, etc. This reagent consists of a mixture of formaldehyde in aqueous solution and concentrated sulfuric acid, which is applied to the suspected substance by drip. Once this is done, the development of different colors reveals the presence of various substances.

• **Symptom:** Subjective evidence of a condition or disease, perceived by the subject suffering from it (e.g., nausea, pain, headache). T. rel. Sign.

• **Psychoactive substance:** chemical substances (drugs or psychotropic drugs) of natural or synthetic origin that affect the functions of the central nervous system (CNS), i.e. the brain and spinal cord. Among their effects, we can find the inhibition of pain, change of mood, alteration of perception, and so on.

• **Self-organization:** Consists of the form of organization and political-social structure that each indigenous people and community gives itself, according to its needs and expectations and according to its traditions and customs.

• **Therapist:** is an individual who has special skills gained through training and experience, either in one or more areas of health care, and whose main task is to provide support to patients who demand it, while the support provided may be of different kinds, usually specialized in a particular area or function and will focus, either with his client or patient, in achieving the goals set.

• **Indigenous Lands:** Lands in which indigenous peoples and communities individually or collectively exercise their original rights and have traditionally and ancestrally developed their physical, cultural, spiritual, social, economic and political life. They include land spaces, areas of cultivation, hunting, fishing, gathering, grazing, settlements, traditional roads, sacred and historical sites, and other areas that they have occupied ancestrally or traditionally and that are necessary to guarantee and develop their specific ways of life.

•   **Toxicity:** Capacity to produce damage to a living organism, in relation to the amount or dose of substance administered or absorbed, the route of administration and its distribution over time (single or repeated doses), type and severity of the damage, time required to produce it, the nature of the organism affected and other intervening conditions.

•   **Toxic: A** substance or physical agent which, acting in very small quantities, is capable of producing adverse effects on living organisms.

•   **Toxicology:** Science that studies chemical substances and physical phenomena insofar as they are capable of producing pathological alterations in living beings, while studying the mechanisms of production of such alterations and the means to counteract them, as well as the procedures to detect, identify and determine such agents and to assess and prevent the risk they represent (mr.).

•   **Forensic Toxicology:** is the branch of toxicology that studies the methods of medico-legal investigation in cases of poisoning and death. Many toxic substances do not generate any characteristic lesion, so that if a toxic reaction is suspected, visual investigation would not be sufficient to reach a conclusion.

•   **Toxification:** Metabolic conversion of a substance into a more toxic one. Ant. detoxification.

•   **Toxin:** Poisonous substance of biological origin, produced by a lower or higher organism of the animal or plant kingdom. The English term toxin is not translatable by toxin but by toxic, of broader meaning. M. gral. Toxic, poison.

•   **Venom:** 1) Animal toxin used for self-defense or predation and usually released by bites or stings. 2) Toxic used intentionally. Syn. p. toxin. Toxic.

•   **Xenobiotic:** strictly speaking, any substance that interacts with an organism and is not one of its natural components. Syn. exogenous substance, foreign substance.

- **Yanomami:** American Indian ethnic group divided into three main groups: Sanumà, Yanomam and Yanam. Although they speak different languages, they understand each other. They are also called *the Yanomami nation*. They live mainly in the state of Amazonas (Venezuela) and in the Brazilian states of Amazonas and Roraima.

Yopo: as *Anadenanthera peregrina* is known, it is a tree from 3 to 18 meters high, with a trunk of 20 to 50 centimeters in diameter and an expanded crown. It is distributed in South America from sea level to 1100 meters of elevation.

Photographic fixations in digital format

Image N° 01

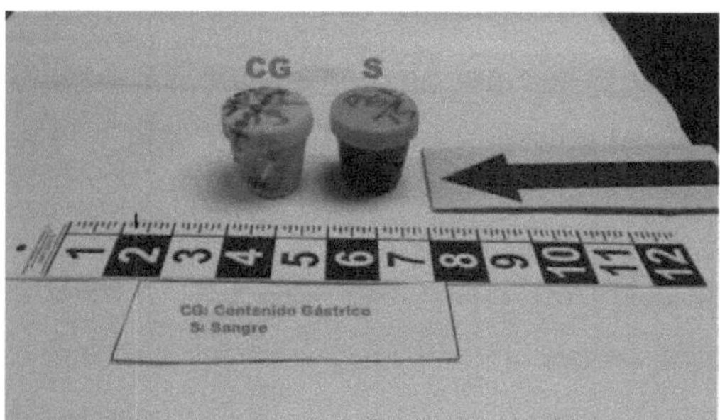

Source: Author's file

Image: This photographic exhibition shows, in general, biological samples, duly collected and preserved.

image 02

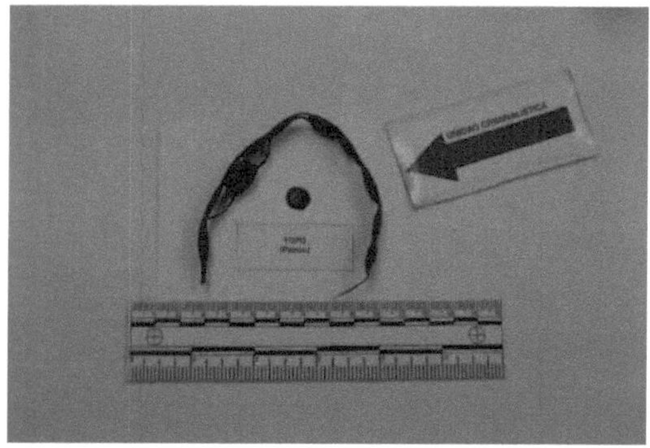

IOW SEMiLLAy

(Source: http://cienciasforenses.mp.gob.ve/toxicologia)

Image 03

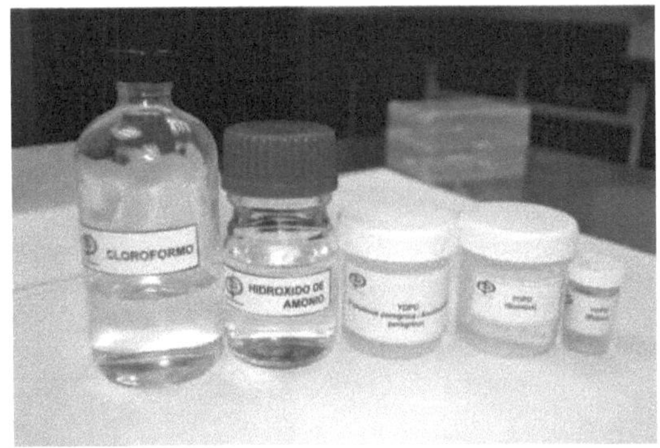

REAGENTS TO BE USED

(Source: http://cienciasforenses.mp.gob.ve/toxicologia)

Image 04

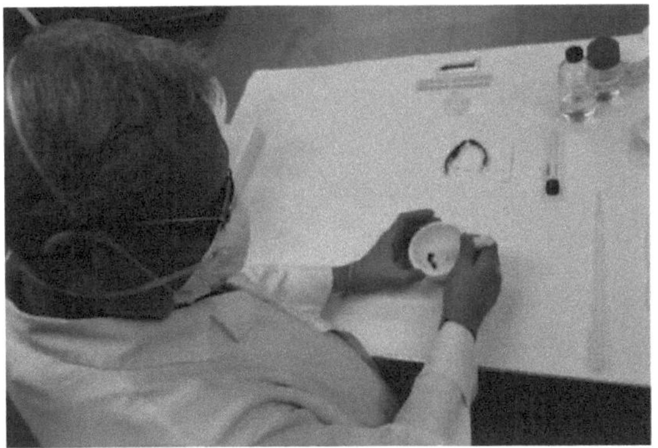

YOPO SPRAYING

(Source: http://cienciasforenses.mp.gob.ve/toxicologia)

Image 05

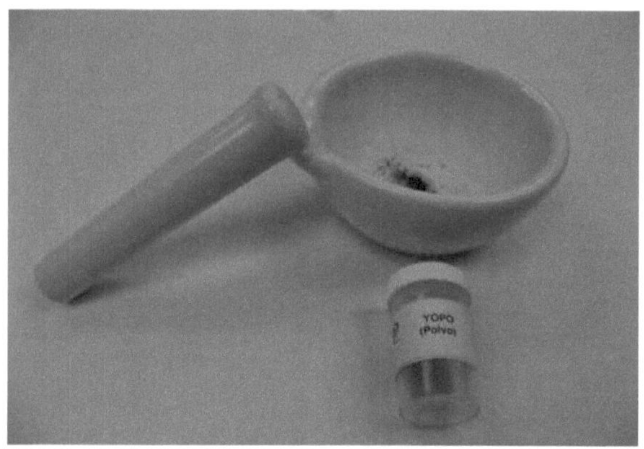

PULVERIZED YOPO SEED

(Source: http://cienciasforenses.mp.gob.ve/toxicologia)

Image 06

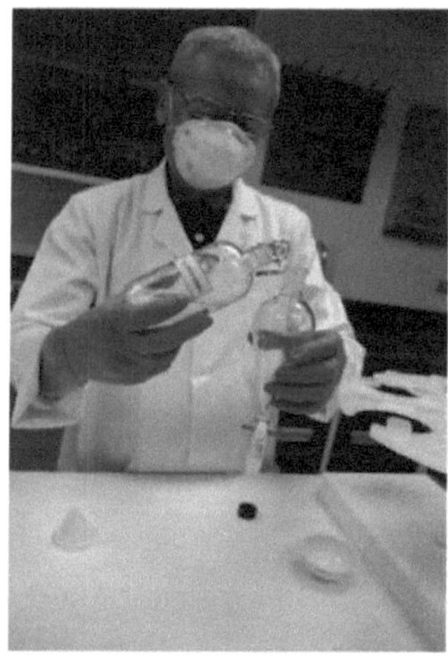

POURING CHLOROFORM 02

(Source: http://cienciasforenses.mp.gob.ve/toxicologia)

Image 07

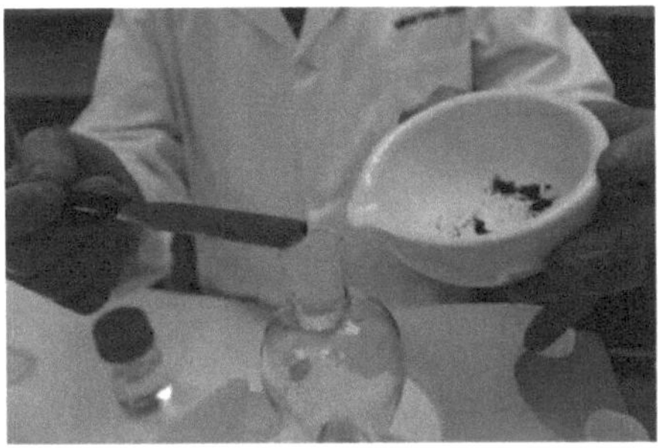

ADDING YOPO POWDER 01

(Source: http://cienciasforenses.mp.gob.ve/toxicologia)

Image 08

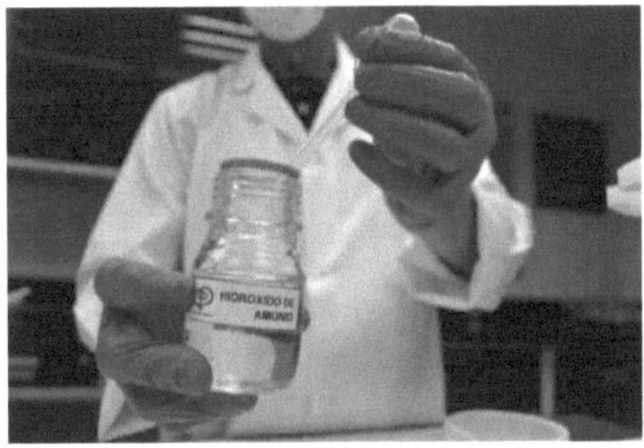

ALKALIZING WITH AMMONIUM HYDROXIDE (DROPS)

(Source: http://cienciasforenses.mp.gob.ve/toxicologia)

Image 09

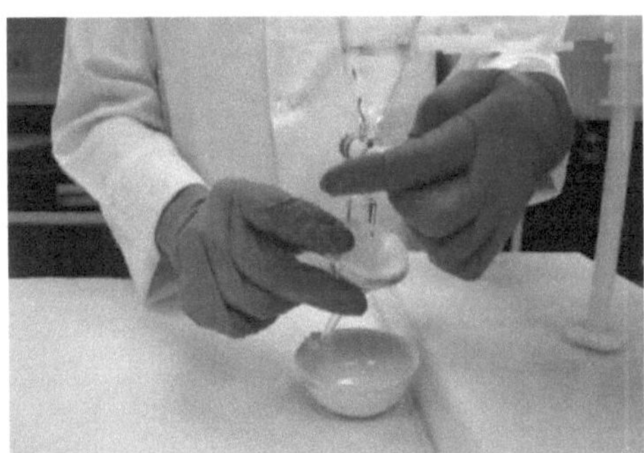

FILTERING THE CHLOROFORMIC PHASE

(Source: http://cienciasforenses.mp.gob.ve/toxicologia)

Image 10

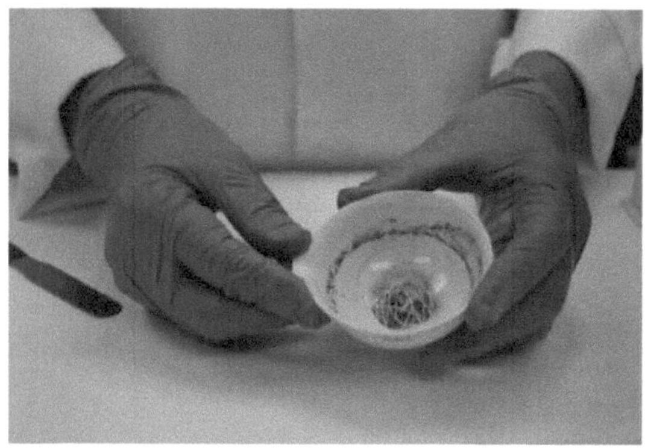

OBTAINING YOPO RESIN

(Source: http://cienciasforenses.mp.gob.ve/toxicologia)

Image 11

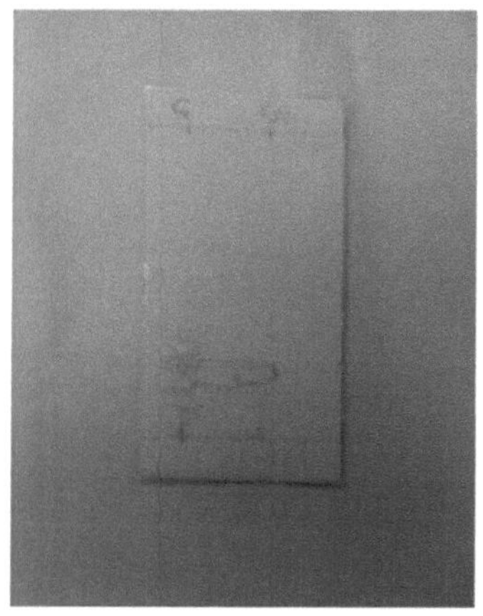

THIN LAYER CHROMATOGRAPHY OF EXTRACT

OF YOPO SEED (Pattern and Sample) WITHOUT DISPLAYER

(Source: Author's Collection)

Image 12

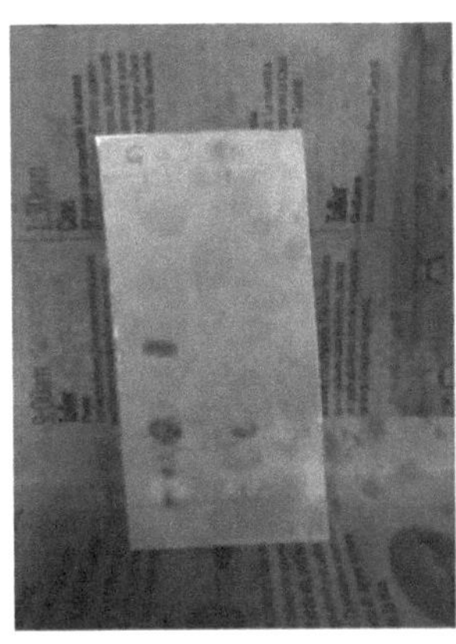

THIN LAYER CHROMATOGRAPHY OF YOPO SEED EXTRACT

(Pattern and Sample) with VISUALIZED (

Source: Author's collection)

Image 13

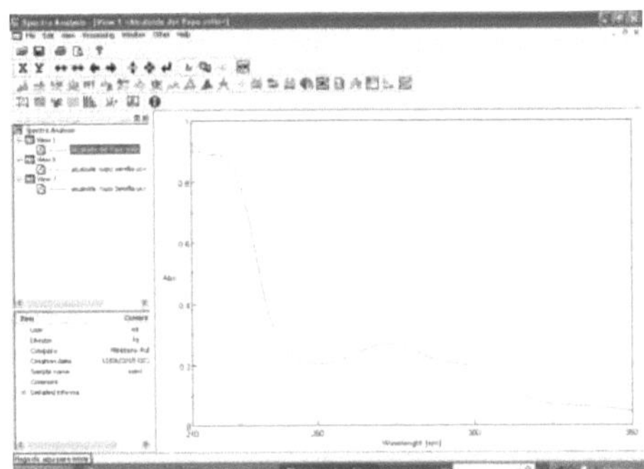

Spectrophotometric curves 01

(YOPO SEED)

(Source: Author's Collection)

IMAGE 14

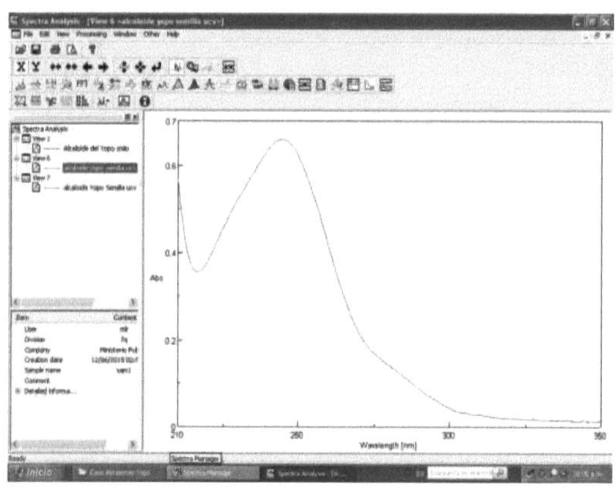

spectrophotometry curves 02

(YOPO SEED MIXTURE) (

Source: Author's file)

IMAGE 15

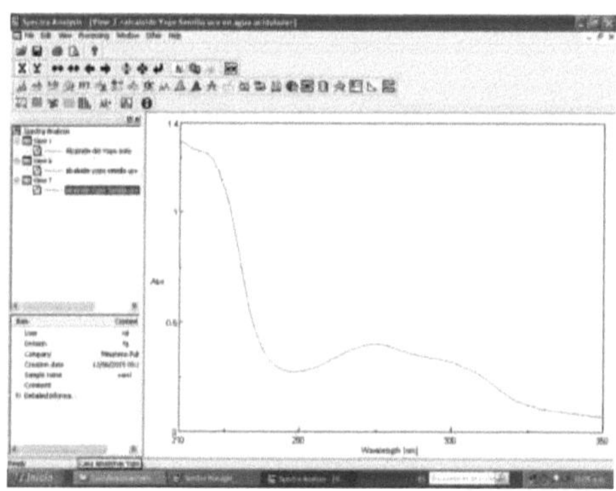

Spectrophotometric curves 03

(YOPO SEED)

(Source: Author's Collection)

IMAGE 16

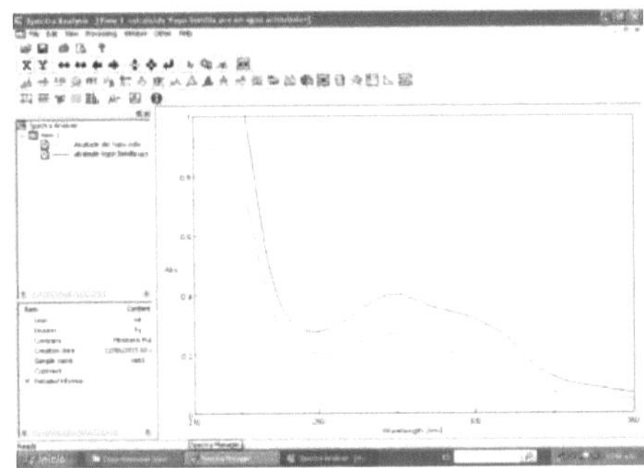

COUPLING OF THE SPECTROPHOTOMETRY CURVES OF THE

YOPO SEED AND YOPO MIXTURE

(Source: Author's Collection)

IMAGE 17

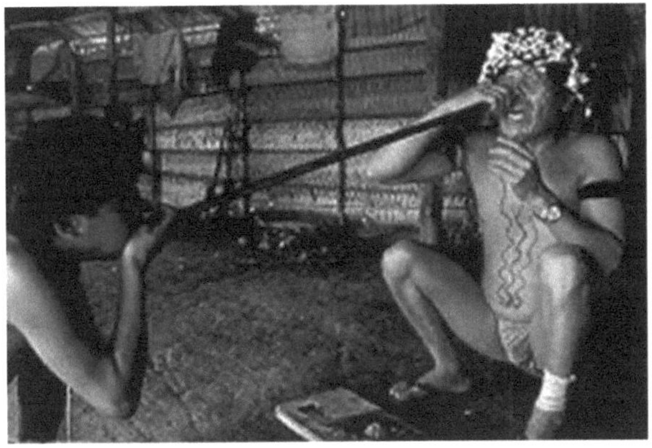

YANOMAMI INDIGENOUS PEOPLE CONSUMING YOPO (
Source: wikipedia)

IMAGE 18

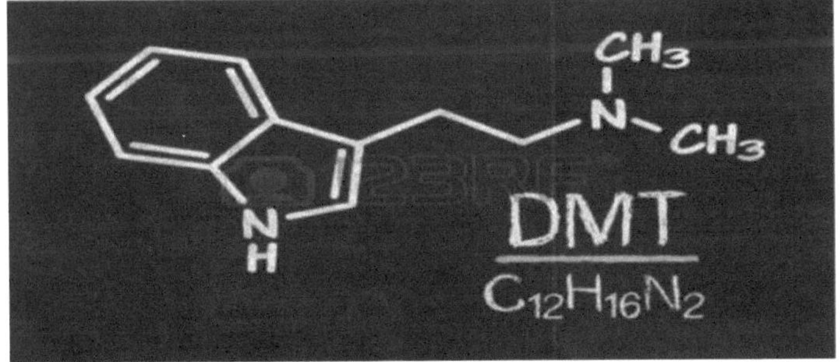

DIMETHYLTRYPTAMINE CHEMICAL FORMULA

(Source: Wikipedia)

Image 19

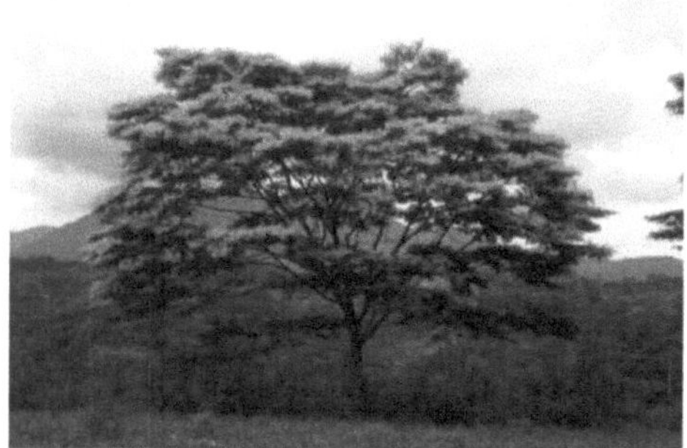

YOPO TREE

(Source: Wikipedia)

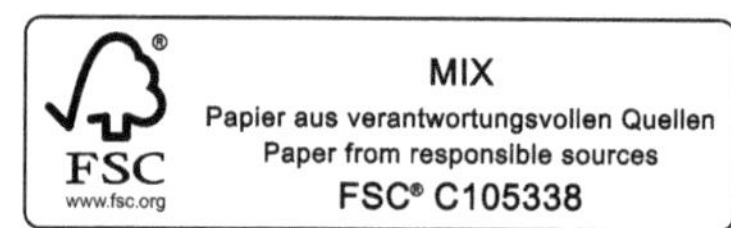

Printed by Books on Demand GmbH, Norderstedt / Germany